Atkins Diet

Rapid Weight Loss Guaranteed

Table of Contents

Introduction 1

Chapter 1: How the Atkins Diet Works 2

Chapter 2: Tremendous Benefits of Eating Low Carb 4

Chapter 3: Atkins and Satiety 7

Chapter 4: Foods You Must Avoid......................................10

Chapter 5: Phases of Atkins 14

Chapter 6: Simple Meals that You Can Start Eating Now.........17

Chapter 7: How Does Weight Loss Work? 21

Chapter 8: Carbs and Sugar..24

Chapter 9: No Sit Ups Required 27

Chapter 10: Why Celebrities Love Atkins............................30

Chapter 11: Why You Don't Need to Count 32

Chapter 12: Atkins Recipes 33

Conclusion..39

Introduction

Congratulations on purchasing your personal copy of *Atkins Diet: Rapid Weight Loss Guaranteed.* Thank you for doing so.

The following chapters will discuss some of the many important benefits of eating a high fat and low carb diet.

You will discover how important it is to make sure that you're getting proper nutrition so that your body can receive the fuel that it needs.

The final chapter will explore many different Atkins recipes.

There are plenty of books on this subject on the market, thanks again for choosing this one! Every effort was made to ensure it is full of as much useful information as possible. Please enjoy!

Chapter 1: How the Atkins Diet Works

Doctor Atkins came up with this diet in response to a need to be able to make sure that people are getting as healthy as possible. He saw so many people who were having trouble with their weight and with the fact that their lifestyle was unhealthy. He wanted to show them that the reason that they were having so many problems with their health was not for any reason other than the large majority of the food that they ate and the fuel they received came directly from carbohydrates. He designed the diet to be able to make sure that people are never left hungry and that they are not only able to lose weight but also that they are able to have a healthy body.

The Atkins diet works by making sure that your body is getting the fuel that it was meant to receive. It focuses on what life would be like without sugar. The diet goes back to the roots of eating when people only had the chance to eat meat and other protein sources along with vegetables. People should not be getting their nutrition from the carbs that most of the people in the United States and other developing countries do – they should be getting it from the fat and protein that comes from animals and other types of sources.

When a person consumes a lot of carbohydrates, they are not converted to fuel in the way that protein and fat are. Instead, they are converted to fat and allowed to sit on the body – your body cannot process carbs in the way that it can process protein and it is not the best source of fuel. While it may last for a short period of time, you will be hungry again within a few hours of eating since the body pushed it through and has already begun turning it into fat.

Aside from the fact that the body was designed specifically for processing protein and other lean sources of fuel, the proof lies in the millions of people who have seen results from the Atkin's diet. These are people who have gone from being morbidly obese to people who are now of a healthy weight – it isn't just about "getting skinny" but is more about allowing the body to function in the most optimal way – the way that it is meant to function.

The diet has been designed to be able to let your body get back to the way that it is supposed to work and give it the best chance at maintaining a healthy weight.

Chapter 2: Tremendous Benefits of Eating Low Carb

There are many benefits that come with eating low carb. Along with the obvious benefits that you will be able to lose detrimental fat off of your body, you will also be able to make sure that you are healthy in other areas. Eating a low carb diet is something that even the trimmest and healthiest of people will be able to benefit from because of the tremendous benefits that it has on the body as a whole. **Low carb eating that is done on the Atkins diet is more of a lifestyle than a typical diet**

Fixed Appetite

Most people in the United States have an appetite that is far out of proportion for what they really need. People no longer eat just to survive and, instead, eat for pleasure, out of social obligations and for other reasons. You need to make sure that your appetite is actually on track with your dietary needs.

A low carb diet is able to do that. It can reduce your appetite in a good way. It will allow you to crave the foods that you *need* instead of just constantly wanting food. It will be a better way for you to eat and you won't have to worry about craving different things. **While following the Atkin's Diet** you'll notice a decrease in appetite. This is the greatest factor that contributes to weight loss.

Abdominal Fat Loss

When you 're eating a low carb diet, you can expect to lose fat from your abdomen first. If you are trying to lose weight, you probably know that this is one of the hardest places to lose fat from so you can take advantage of it just happening naturally from consuming a reduced number of carbs. This is beneficial even for people who do not need to lose a lot of weight – everyone has a small amount of fat that is around their abdomen. It really wouldn't hurt anyone to lose a little weight from that area because of the benefits that come from it. By eating low carbs, you can make sure that you are getting the best belly fat reduction possible.

Higher HDL

While we tend to think of cholesterol as a bad thing, the bad type is only one of the two kinds. It comes from eating an unhealthy diet and is made in response to the bad food that you are eating. There is actually good cholesterol and your body needs to have it. The good type of cholesterol is called HDL and it can actually help you to lose more weight and maintain a healthier lifestyle. Eating low carbs will help to decrease the bad cholesterol and increase the good kind so that you can make sure that you are getting the most and losing the most amount of weight possible. This is important if you want to make sure that you are going to be able to maintain a healthy lifestyle along with losing weight.

Better Blood Sugar

Unsurprisingly, eating a lot of foods that are high in carbs (sugar) actually raises your blood sugar. High blood sugar can lead to a host of problems that can cause you to be unhealthy. From metabolic disorder to diabetes and all other types of nutrition-based diseases, high blood sugar is downright bad for your health. Eating a diet that is protein and fat rich with very reduced amounts of sugar (and carbs) will allow you to decrease your blood sugar to normal, healthy levels.

Metabolic Syndrome

The Atkins diet is not a cure for any type of disease and was never intended to be anything other than a way for people to reduce their weight and help with their obesity but it has been shown to help people who have metabolic syndrome. This is a problem where the metabolism does not perform in the way that it should and it can be combatted by eating a healthier diet. It is important that you know that if you have metabolic syndrome or any disease, you should talk with your doctor before trying any type of diet plan.

Therapeutic for Disorders

Even though the Atkins diet is not a cure for diseases, it can be very therapeutic for people who have a plethora of different disorders. This can help everything from brain disorders, mood disorders and other things that are detrimental to your health. There are many other things that you can help yourself feel better with when you are eating in a healthy way with low carbs and following the Atkins diet.

Weight Loss

The biggest benefit, and the one that the Atkins Diet is always aiming to help with, is the weight loss that you will see from eating reduced carbs. This is the number one reason that the people who diet choose to go on this diet and you can make sure that you are going to be able to enjoy the diet and the weight loss benefits that come from it. By following the diet, you will be able to lose weight – whether you need to lose 30 pounds or 300 – the diet is a way that you can change your eating habits for the better.

Chapter 3: Atkins and Satiety

People who do the Atkins diet have been shown to be more satisfied than people who eat the traditional low-fat high carbohydrate diets that have been used for decades. The diet allows people to remain full for two reasons. The first is that people who are doing Atkins are able to make sure that they are eating any time that they are hungry – they are not restricted in the number of calories. The second reason is that they are eating a lot of protein. They can benefit from this because it takes the body much longer to process protein into fuel and they will be able to make sure that they are getting the most from the diet. Since it takes the body longer to process protein and it is harder, they will remain fuller for a long time.

At the Beginning

Many people who start a diet think that they will have to stop eating all of the things that they love to eat when they start the diet. That is not the case, though, with the Atkins diet. You can still enjoy hamburgers, bacon and even your favorite vegetables as long as you do the diet the right way. You should make sure that you are able to eat the things that you want and that you are getting plenty of protein and fat, especially in the beginning.

When you first start out, you can be sure that you are always as full as possible and that you are going to be satisfied with all of the food that you eat. The food that you eat will be filling since you can, essentially, eat until you are full. You can also eat often when you are doing the Atkins diet.

It is actually suggested that you eat around six small meals every day when you are doing the diet instead of eating the typical three large meals. This means that you will need to be prepared to eat more food. The more fat and protein that you consume, the more satisfied you will be. This will help you to make sure that you are going to be able to truly do the diet in the right way. It is a good idea to make sure that you are getting the most fuel possible and that you will be able to use it up. The Atkins diet is designed in a way that allows you to eat what you need to.

Dieters who are able to feel satisfied and who do not have to worry about skipping meals or drastically cutting down the amount of food that they are eating will be more successful on the diet that they are doing. When you are doing Atkins, you are encouraged to eat as much as it takes you to feel full and that will help you to be as successful as possible on the diet. You can even eat more than you typically would and still lose weight because you are not eating carbs that build up fat around your stomach and other areas of your body.

Since you will be eating until you are full, there will be less of a chance of you stopping the diet. Even if you are not eating carbs, you will still feel as full as possible when you eat because of the meals that you are eating and because you will be eating more often. It is an ideal diet for people who struggle with overeating.

You will even be able to find that, the more that you do the Atkins diet, the less you will need to eat to be able to stay full. This may seem counterintuitive because you are actually eating more but the diet works in a way that allows your body to understand that it is getting the nourishment that it needs. You need to make sure that you are eating enough to feel full even if the end game is to be able to eat less. Your body will adjust as necessary when it is getting the right type of nutrition so that you don't need to worry about trying to change your eating habits...aside from cutting carbs, of course.

Protein as Fuel

When you are doing the Atkins diet, the fuel that you get will all come from protein. Even when you are eating fat, you are actually getting a decent amount of protein from that. Your body is going to be powered by the protein instead of powered by the carbs that you are used to. It will be able to use the protein as a clean fuel for your body which will enable you to make sure that you are getting the most from the diet. It is among the best options for people who need to be able to stay full but who want to stop gaining weight.

The way that protein works to make you fuller for longer is that it takes longer for the body to process it. The body will need to go through a longer process once the food enters your stomach. It will need to work harder to be able to turn it to energy and that takes a much longer time than if you were just eating carbs that are burned off very quickly. The protein is not burned quickly and will, for that reason, keep you fuller for longer.

As your body gets used to using protein as fuel, you will need less and less of it until you are at a healthy eating place. The body was designed to be able to adapt and it will be able to run on autopilot once you make sure that you are getting the most out of it. It will also be much easier for you to make sure that you are getting the best experience out of the diet when you can stick with it through all of the phases that allow you to make sure that you are going to be able to lose weight and get healthy.

Chapter 4: Foods You Must Avoid

To make sure that Atkins works, you will need to avoid certain foods. While some of these foods are traditionally thought of as unhealthy, some of them have long been touted as health foods. You will find that even these supposed health foods have negative effects on your health especially when you are trying to eat a low carb diet. This is something that you need to make sure that you are doing so that you are not able to continue gaining weight.

While many diets have a small amount of wiggle room that you can use if you want to be able to "cheat" on the diet, there is no room for that with Atkins. This is due to two major reasons. The first reason is that you're actually allowed to eat many different kinds of foods on the diet – there is no need for you to cheat on it since you can still enjoy a lot of your favorite foods. The second reason is that you will ruin the science of the diet. The diet is backed by the chemistry of the body and involves a process that the body is able to enter into. If you cheat, you will take the body out of it and you will have to start over. For that reason, you should try your best not to "cheat" at Atkins especially when you are first getting started. That is, unless you want to start the whole process over again which really isn't a healthy idea for anyone especially someone who has a lot of weight that they need to lose.

The idea behind Atkins is that you don't eat any carbohydrates. Carbs can be found in things like bread and pasta, but did you know that you can actually find carbs in other places that are hidden, like in your favorite potato vegetables and even in some things like processed foods where carbs are hidden because the companies that create them use sugar as a way to make sure that the foods taste good and are able to be preserved for a long time. Watch out for hidden carbs and if you find anything in the ingredients that looks like sugar (lose, tose, ose endings).

This is not a complete list of foods that you should avoid but it does cover some of the major ones that you will come across while you are dieting:

Artificial sweeteners (limit these) – while these don't necessarily have sugar in them, you should try to avoid them because the artificial sugar can make you crave real sugar

Bananas – with the highest fruit carb count, avoid bananas at all costs!

Beans – even though these have a lot of protein in them, they still contain a lot of carbs it is especially important to avoid them in the first two phases of Atkins

Beer – this has long been called the bread of drinks – it has as much yeast in it as bread and often has the same (or more) carbs

Berries – while these are the *lowest* carb count fruits you can eat, they still have a lot of carbs and can contribute to belly fat

Bread (any kind) – this is the most obvious of all of the things that you should avoid, bread is filled with carbs

Buns – even the so-called "health" versions (like brioche, etc) are not great

Cakes – packed with sugar in its pure form *and* carbs from the flour

Cereal – even "bran" cereals that would normally be considered healthy are not safe if you're avoiding carbs

Chocolate – even just a nibble of chocolate can have addictive effects

Couscous – some diets allow for whole grain (or brown couscous). Atkins does not

French fries – the snack version of potatoes – avoid them

Hot cereal – everything from oatmeal to grits is filled with carbs

Ice cream – while the protein count is great thanks to the milk used in ice cream, it's not worth the sugar

Lentils – similar to beans and should be avoided when you are first getting started, only small amounts after you have completed the diet

Margarine – with all of the processed ingredients in this, the carbs add up and can make it harder for you to achieve your weight loss goals

Most alcoholic beverages – the majority of alcoholic beverages have a lot of carbs in them – avoid them especially in the first stages

Most fruit – most of the fruit, save for things like tomatoes, have a lot of carbs in them avoid them while you are doing the Atkins diet

Muesli – this is a carb-ridden food

Oatmeal – like other hot cereals, oatmeal should be avoided

Other fake butter – similar to margarine, imitation butter has a lot of carbs. Stick with the real sticks and you will be fine – the fat content of real butter will also help you to stay fuller for longer

Pasta – the noodle of bread! avoid this unless you find a carb free egg version

Pastries – these are similar to other desserts and can be packed with even hidden sugar

Porridge – even though this is a comforting hot food, it is loaded with carbs

Potato chips – try to stay away from these even though they can be tempting – a great alternative is pork rinds that you can dip in your favorite chip dips

Potatoes – starchy vegetables and fruits are generally not your friend when you are doing a low carb diet

Quinoa – this ancient grain is still a grain and, as such, should be avoided while you are doing Atkins

Rice – even brown rice has carbs in it, stay away from this

Soft drinks – even diet soft drinks are not great for you even though they don't have carbs

Sports drinks – touted as healthy, are not even close because they have high sugar content

Sugar – all of the rest of the foods to avoid include sugar and byproducts of sugar

Sweet potatoes – despite the health benefits that come with sweet potatoes, they are a starch vegetable just like potatoes are

Tortillas – even though they are sometimes labeled low carb, they still have a lot of carbs in them

Wine – the fruit content in this raises the sugar in it and causes it to have a lot of carbs

Chapter 5: Phases of Atkins

Like many other diets that most people are able to do, the Atkins diet has different steps to it. These are known as the phases and you will go through each of these phases when you decide to do the diet. It is a good idea to follow the phases exactly like they are set up to be done so that you can lose the most amount of weight possible and get the biggest benefit out of the diet.

Phase 1

This is the first two weeks of your diet. It is the time when you will learn all about low carb and you will kick start what you are going to be losing in the future. Try to make sure that you are keeping your carb count to under 20 grams per day. These should come from <1-3 grams of carbs in each of your foods (for example, cheese may have 1 or 2 carbs in it).

You should be eating very high protein and very high fat during this time. There really shouldn't be many carbs at all. You may even need to avoid most vegetables during this time. Aside from green leafy vegetables, most of the ones have more than a few carbs in them. You should only do this for about two weeks of the diet.

Phase 2

During this phase of the diet, you will learn to eat low carb with just a little more carbs added back in. This is where you will spend the longest time at while you are doing Atkins. It should only be done after you have entered ketosis through stage one and will be the point where you will stay until you get close to your goal weight.

During this point, you can add things like milk and nuts back into your diet. You can also add vegetables (except for potatoes) back into your diet. If you would like to add fruit back at this time, you can start eating berries but be careful not to eat too many because this can cause you to start gaining weight again.

Phase 3

You should only enter this phase after you have made it through phase 2 and are getting very close to the weight where you want to be. This is how you stop the weight loss process of your diet. You can add back nearly all of the fruits to your diet during this time. This is also where you will add beans back.

The phase 3 can take anywhere from a few weeks to a few months depending on how long it takes for you to stop those weight loss hormones. You need to make sure that you are adding back enough so that you won't continue to lose weight. There is a point that you will need to find – for this reason, it is called the fine-tuning phase. You don't want to add too many or too few carbs to your diet. It is all about trying different things during this phase to see what works.

Phase 4

You can maintain your weight for the rest of your life by staying in phase 4. You should be eating healthy carbs like beans, nuts and even some whole grain breads. You can eat these but it should be in moderation. You need to watch very closely what you are eating. If you find that you are starting to gain weight back, drop back down to the amount of carbs that you were eating in phase 3.

The best thing about maintenance is that the longer you are in this phase for, the easier it will be to stay in it. You need to make sure that you are watching always but you should also let your guard down a little bit. As you learn what carbs you can eat without gaining weight and what you can do with the carbs that you have eaten, you will get better at maintenance.

It is very easy to fix any mistakes that you may have made while you were maintaining your carb free lifestyle. You can just stop eating the carbs that you were eating before and it should not take very long to be able to get back to where you were at. Just be sure to not let your carb eating or your weight get too far out of control.

Importance of Phases

The idea behind the Atkins diet is that you enter into what is known as ketosis. This is where your body starts to use the fat that is stored upon your body instead of using the food that you are eating for fuel. It is a point that does take some work to get to but is very efficient at shedding the pounds when you actually get to that point. If you start to eat carbs again – even if you just eat one piece of bread – you will not be in ketosis anymore. It is a bad idea to do this because you will have to start out the process again with the induction phase and put yourself into ketosis again.

If you do not follow the phases exactly how they are outlined, you will not have the chance to lose all of the weight that you could be losing. This also means that you will not have the healthiest body possible – following the phases exactly as they are supposed to be followed will allow you to make the healthiest decisions and will give you a chance to make sure that you are getting the most out of the diet and everything that you are going to be able to do with the diet.

Chapter 6: Simple Meals that You Can Start Eating Now

You don't have to do the most complex or complicated recipes to be able to get the most out of Atkins. Simple switches to your normal eating habits will allow you to truly get the most out of the diet and can be easy enough that you can start right away. Each of these is *simple* meal ideas that do not require a complicated recipe – try them out, tweak them and enjoy them for each of your meals!

Breakfast Ideas

- Omelet with cheddar, fried onions, and mushrooms
- Scrambled eggs with Colby jack cheese – be sure to fry in butter
- Eggs benedict with *no* English muffin (the whole recipe is carb free when you take out the English muffin)
- Green peppers and eggs (sauté the green peppers in butter to get the most flavor out of them or switch them out for hot peppers if you want a zing that will really kick you into action in the morning)
- Eggs, chopped ham, and feta cheese
- Eggs with cream cheese, spinach and artichoke hearts
- Bacon
- Eggs with chopped bacon and cheddar cheese
- Denver omelet (eggs, bacon and green peppers topped with onion and cheddar cheese cooked in a large pan)
- Muffins made out of a combination equal of eggs and cottage cheese
- Add some plain Greek yogurt to your eggs to give them a better texture
- Swap out the butter for coconut oil if you don't have it or if you just want to do something different
- Add *any* type of meat to your eggs
- Add *any* type of cheese to your eggs
- Consider spinach and kale to add to your eggs for a leafy green crunch

Lunch Ideas

- Salami and cream cheese rolled up
- Ham and swiss rolled up
- Turkey and cheddar rolled up
- Mix and match each of these
- A salad with all of your favorite vegetables
- Visit Chipotle and ask for everything in a bowl – avoid rice, avoid beans if you are in phase 1
- Grilled chicken from *any* fast food
- Hamburgers no bun from any fast food
- Avocado, tomato, mozzarella, boiled egg with balsamic (avocado Caprese salad)
- Shrimp stir fried with cauliflower make sure not to add any rice to it and only vegetables that are not starchy
- Shawarma from your favorite Indian restaurant
- Beef and broccoli (ask for no rice so you aren't tempted) from a reputable Chinese restaurant
- Lettuce laid flat with avocado, tomato, turkey, bacon and ranch dressing on them
- Zucchini fried in butter and tomatoes with chopped boiled eggs to it
- Brunch foods like eggs and bacon
- Cauliflower chopped into small pieces like rice and put into any dish or simply eaten on its own with a little bit of salt and pepper (or bacon and cheese)
- Mexican corn dip (corn, cheese, mayonnaise, pico de gallo)
- An egg baked into an avocado and topped with tomatoes
- Chicken breast that is coated in parmesan cheese (for crunch) and baked

Dinner Ideas

- Spaghetti squash – be sure to use a sauce that does not have a lot of carbs in it or (ideally) any. You can make your own sauce easily with some tomato paste and a combination of your favorite spices
- Pot roast (use carrots instead of potatoes) – add onions along with celery for the best flavor possible

- "Un" sandwiches – lettuce rolled up with your favorite sandwich fillings in them
- Open faced burgers – grill and top your burgers like you normally would except don't put them on a bun
- Steak – try different ways of cooking it, doing it in the pan with butter and olive oil is great but so is grilling it on the grill. Add asparagus or steamed broccoli for a delicious side
- Any fish that is cooked to the Atkins standards (meaning, don't bread it). Shrimp is also great with cocktail sauce just be sure that you get the kind that doesn't have a whole lot of sugar in it
- Grilled chicken is great any way that you make it. Rub it with garam masala for a Middle Eastern twist. Put Cajun rub on it for a spice that you won't believe. Simply add some seasoning salt to the breasts for a simple meal that you will be able to eat anytime. You can also save some of the chicken back for later and top salads, eggs and anything else that you want with it. Chicken salad anyone?
- Any casserole that you have a recipe for, just eliminate the rice, noodles or other carbs so that you can continue the Atkins diet. You can also substitute it for the cauliflower rice that we talked about earlier on in this recipe. Cauliflower makes a great substitution in casseroles and many people will not even notice the difference because cauliflower doesn't have too much flavor on its own

Snack Ideas

- Chicken salad – if you like chicken salad spread, make a big bowl of it at the beginning of the week. You can eat it on its own when you are hungry, put it in a lettuce wrap or design a lunch around it
- Egg salad – even easier to snack on than chicken salad, store this in the fridge for up to one week
- Pickles – just be sure you don't get the sweet kind because they have sugar in them. Dill pickles are great when you are craving carbs or are hungry. The crunch helps to satisfy you and the salt gives you the boost that

you need to keep the day going

- Boiled eggs – you can use these for recipes or you can simply keep them handy. If you are going to save some for snacks, be sure that you store them in some water in a sealed container so that you can make sure they don't get too dry
- Pork rinds – if you are a chip eater, these will be your perfect snack. They come in many different flavors but you can also eat them with your favorite dip (as long as it is carb free)

Chapter 7: How Does Weight Loss Work?

Weight loss doesn't just happen because you are eating healthier. It is a scientific process that happens as a result of years of evolution and what the body was designed to be able to do – survive. It is not necessary to know how weight loss works to be able to achieve it but having an idea of the way that your body works to lose weight will allow you to better understand the way that it works. It will also allow you to have an easier time at making sure you are doing all of the right things on the diet.

Why We Gain Weight

All humans gain weight at some point in their lives. Whether you are overweight or obese or you are of a healthy weight, the chances are that you gained weight at some point in your life (unless, of course, you are an 8-pound baby reading this book). The point of gaining weight is so that you are able to survive. If you didn't have *any* fat, you wouldn't be able to stay warm, you wouldn't be able to be protected in the event that you fell down or you ran into something and you wouldn't be able to truly live your life in the way that humans are meant to be able to live. Making sure that you are able to gain weight is important and a key part of evolution. Thousands of years ago, the Paleolithic people needed to gain weight in the winter to be able to keep themselves warm and then shed it in the summer because they were active and eating buffalo and things like that.

How We Lose Weight

People lose weight one of two ways: through a drastic reduction in the type of food that they are eating (caloric deficit) or through a change in the way that the body processes food (like ketosis). You can restrict your calories and you will most definitely lose weight but it could take some time. The easiest way for you to make sure that you are actually losing weight in the fastest way possible is to change the way that your body is able to process food and change it to fuel (or use its own resources for fuel).

Your Body Eats Your Fat

The easiest way to explain how you can lose weight with Atkins is that your body is eating its own fat. Since you are not giving it the carbs that are easy to process, digest and turn into fuel, you will need to allow the body the time that it needs to be able to process protein but it sometimes needs that fuel while it is still processing the protein. That is where the fat inside of your body comes into play. Your body will process that "fuel" you have stored up (AKA your muffin top) to be able to give you the energy that you need. This is what happens when you starve in a literal sense but Atkins isn't actually starving yourself, it is just you being able to use the process to your benefit.

Understanding Your Body's Needs

The thing is, though, that you can't really live off of the fat that you have (even if you have a lot). Even people who are very obese would eventually die from starvation if they were not eating anything. It is important, for this reason, that you continue to eat while you are doing Atkins. The only thing that you need to worry about is eating a lot of protein and fat. Your body will be able to stay alive (obviously) and it will do all of the hard work that comes with processing the protein and using your fat to stay alive.

Weight Loss Hormones Come On

Once your body realizes that it isn't starving and that something different is going on, the adrenal system will take a step back and will realize that what you are doing is *good*. It will tell the rest of the body to stop storing that fat and to let it go. The fat will eventually come out of the places where it is stored and then it can be used for fuel.

But Where Does that Fat Go?

You don't have to worry about where the fat goes because you will just know that it is leaving your stomach, your thighs, and your backside. If you really are interested, though, it is actually turned into carbon and released from the body through your breath. While most people think that they are excreting fat because they use the bathroom a lot more while losing weight, only a very small percentage of your fat comes out of your body through your excretions. It is converted to energy through anaerobic activity and then transformed into carbon and simply breathed out of your body.

Gaining it Back

Gaining weight back can be even more detrimental than the first time that you had it on your body. This is why yo-yo dieting is such a bad idea. Your body gets used to the lose-gain-rinse-repeat cycle. It will become immune to your weight loss efforts. It is best to get Atkins right on the first try and follow each of the four stages for the rest of your life so that you don't have to worry about that cycle kicking in.

Carbs Kill Survival

People weren't necessarily meant to eat all of the carbs that they currently do. They also weren't created to sit for 10 hours per day or have multiple stressors in the way that they do, but it is all part of modern life. There are a few things that you, as a human, can do to make sure that you are surviving optimally. Avoiding carbs is one of the biggest things that you can do and your body will thank you for being able to do it. You will also have far less stress and you will be healthier even if you sit for long periods of time after you have lost the weight that you need to lose.

Chapter 8: Carbs and Sugar

Sugar is bad for the body – nearly everyone can agree with that fact. It is:

- Toxic
- Addictive
- Corrosive
- Damaging to every system of the body

The problem with sugar, though, is that it is in so many hidden places that the chances of you finding it even in the most ordinary situations are very slim. You need to make sure that you know what is going on with sugar, how it can affect you and the different problems that come along with sugar. It is also important to make sure that you know that sugar is bad for you and that you are going to be able to get rid of sugar. When you are starting a low carb diet like Atkins, it can be very easy to sink back into the sugar trap because of how hard it is to cut sugar out of your life but you need to make sure that you are not falling back into that trap and that you are fighting the withdrawals that come along with sugar.

Addictive Sugar and Atkins Flu

When you are first starting Atkins, you may notice that you start to feel like you might have the flu. Some people even develop symptoms that are so bad that they are stuck in bed for a day or more. Many mistake this for the flu, though and chalk it up to coincidence. Some people stop their diet thinking that they are doing the right thing by feeding the flu to try to get rid of it, but this is actually a bad idea.

What people are going through is what is known affectionately as the Atkins flu. It is not a real condition and it is not related to the actual influenza in any way, but some people call it that because they realize that the diet is what is making them not feel good. Don't stop the diet, though, because it is all a part of the process of starting Atkins and learning the right way to eat.

What people are actually going through is simply withdrawal

symptoms. When you drop from eating a lot of sugar to eating none or very, very little sugar, you will start to enter a withdrawal. Similar to what drug addicts go through, your body is learning how to compensate without the sugar that you have been funneling down your throat throughout your entire life. It is a good thing and something that many people must go through while they are switching to low carb.

The number one thing that you *must* do to make sure that you are not going to ruin your diet is do not start eating carbs again. Stay off of the carbs and work your way through the withdrawals so that you can make sure that you are going to be able to continue with the diet. It is so important that you do everything that you can to make sure that you are going to be able to get the most out of the diet and that you are not going to get into any problems that come along with Atkins and the low-carb lifestyle.

Sugar's Bad, What About Bread?

Now that we know about sugar, it should be fine to eat bread and noodles because they're not sweet, right? Wrong!

Bread and noodles don't necessarily have sugar in them in the way that you would normally think about it (they're not sweet) but they do have carbs. When your body takes carbs in, it is not able to digest them in the way that they are and it certainly cannot turn them into fuel in their pure form. Instead, it takes the carbs, turns them into sugar through the processes in the body and then uses them for fuel.

Sugar as a fuel is really not great, though. Think about burning sugar – it gets hot, burns, and is gone in just a few seconds. It burns like that in your body too. It is used up very quickly and you are left wandering around looking for your next sugar fix. To make sure that you are getting long lasting fuel, you need to find something that is somewhat difficult for you to digest and for your body to process into fuel – protein!

So, just because bread is not sweet doesn't mean that it isn't sugar. The carbs are basically sugar and that is just as harmful to your health as all of the other sugary things that you have been eating for your whole life.

Watch for Hidden Sugar

Another way that people go wrong when they are doing the Atkins diet is with hidden sugar. This is the sugar that they do not think about. The sugar that hides in a can of green beans, is in your favorite pork rinds or even your spices. Sugar is everywhere and it is used in things that you use every day even though it is not even really necessary. Fast food companies are very well known for sneaking hidden sugar into things and, for that reason, you should avoid even low carb fast food options if it is anything that you can avoid.

When you are doing Atkins, you need to read labels and try to find everything out about the foods that you are eating when you are eating them so that you don't accidentally consume hidden sugars. Be vigilant about your sugar search and if you find something that has sugar in it, take it out of your diet. You don't need that in your life and you will not be able to really get the benefits of the diet if you are still consuming secret sugars (even if you *are* losing weight – it is still harmful to your health).

Chapter 9: No Sit Ups Required

There are quite a few benefits that come with the Atkins diet. Not only will you be able to lose weight on it in a much shorter time than from simply cutting calories but you will also notice that it is one of the most comfortable diets to do. Aside from the brief sugar addiction problems that you will go through at the beginning (which usually only last a few days), you will be able to truly feel like you are not wanting for anything when it comes to Atkins.

No Exercise Needed

Losing weight with no exercise required sounds like a dream to many people but that is exactly what Atkins is. You don't have to worry about exercising when you are doing the diet because the results that you are getting from your eating habits alone are just as beneficial as the results that you would be getting from diet and exercise on any other diet. It is a great way for you to be able to lose weight even if you are unable to exercise.

Phase 2

While some people may want to still exercise while they are doing Atkins, it is actually suggested that you wait until you are in, at least, phase 2 before you start exercising. This will allow your body to enter ketosis and to start making the switches that it needs to make before you try to add exercising to your routine.

Since the idea of ketosis is such a delicate balance, you need to make sure that you are not going to upset it in any way. Adding exercise in too early could do this and you may not be able to get the results that you want. You may also start building up a lot of muscle from exercising. While muscle is great for burning fat, it can affect the number that you see on your scale since it does weigh you down.

Make sure that you are only exercising when you are in phase 2 and not doing it too early. You want to make sure that you are truly going to be able to get the most out of Atkins and exercising could truly compromise that if you don't know the right way to do it or you simply don't want to be able to do it.

Fullness in Diet

Diets often fail because people are hungry. When you are hungry, you may tend to reach for the first thing that you find – even if it is filled with carbs. You should make sure that you are trying to stay as full as possible at all times and that you are going to be able to always make the right choices with the food that you are reaching for whether it is a snack or some other meal. There are many different techniques that you can do to make sure that you are not going to fall back into the trap of unhealthy eating.

With Atkins, the chances are that you will probably never be that hungry. This is because you can essentially have anything that you want to eat as long as it is carb free at any time. There is no strict schedule for eating or times where you are restricted. If you're hungry, all you need to do is eat something and as long as it doesn't have carbs in it, you won't mess up the progress that you have made with your weight loss and the things that you have done.

Things You Can Have

Since there are so few things that you can't have, you should not ever feel like you are restricted. You can eat all of the foods that you love – bacon, steak, even cheese – and you will still lose weight. Atkins is one of the easiest diets that you can do because it allows you to eat food that you love, make minor tweaks to your diet and still see huge results on the scale with the way that you are working to make sure that you are losing weight.

It is also a great way for you to lose weight because you can still eat out, visit fast food restaurants and you don't have to work too hard to make special meals for yourself that are separate from what you would normally feed your family – just change the recipe around a bit to be carb free and everyone can enjoy the same meal.

Atkins was designed so that people would be able to be successful with weight loss and when you do it, you will have the chance at being successful and also being able to eat all of the things that you have already loved – no diet food here!

Even the Drinks

Another nice factor that was added into Atkins is that even tea and coffee drinkers don't have to make major switches to the drinks that they consume. This is nice because you will be able to still enjoy your tea, coffee and diet soda while you are doing Atkins. As long as there is no added sugar in each of these things, you will be able to still enjoy them.

While diet soda does have an artificial sweetener in it, it is still something that you can enjoy while you are doing Atkins. You may find that your sugar habit is harder to quit when you are drinking diet soda and you may also find that you are not getting the best results as quickly but that is sometimes worth it for people to be able to have the diet soda that they love so much in their lives. Consider making a switch later on from diet soda to tea or coffee with just creamer in it because there are a lot of negative health problems that can come from drinking diet soda all of the time – tea and coffee have their own, too but they are far less than diet soda problems.

Chapter 10: Why Celebrities Love Atkins

As a diet that has been hailed one of the best by mega-celebrity Kim Kardashian and has many followers in Hollywood, Atkins is something that even the famous people can get behind because of the way that it works. There are many benefits that come along with Atkins as we have already learned about but what is it that makes Atkins such an attractive option for people who are living the high life as celebrities? Here, we'll see some of the reasons that celebrities love the diet and why you should, too.

It is Easy

A diet that you can still eat your favorite foods on is something that even celebrities can get behind. The Atkins diet does not require you to count complicated points or figure out your calorie to fat and protein ratios. Instead, it simply says – don't eat carbs! That's it. The diet is so easy that anyone can understand it and apply it.

There isn't really any prep work that is involved with Atkins other than stocking up on snacks and other low carb foods while getting rid of the food that you have in your house that could be a trigger. For this reason, celebrities love it. They could need to lose a ton of weight with just a very short notice so they try to do Atkins because of the way that it allows them to simply switch their eating habits and make them their own in a short period of time.

It is for Busy Lives

Since the diet was designed for real people, it is perfect for those who lead busy lives and who is busier than celebrities? Whether they are schlepping to their next appearance or trying to promote themselves, they lead very busy lives. For that reason, they are able to take advantage of Atkins and get all of the benefits that come along with it. It is something that they are able to do in the best way and something that makes it better for them.

When celebrities do a diet, they need to make sure that they are going to be able to do every aspect of the diet. With Atkins, the only thing that they have to worry about is eating no carbs. They don't have to do extra exercises or anything like that which could take more precious time away from what they already have. It is important to note that celebrities are just as busy, if not busier, than average people so they need to have a diet that works for them. Those who are on the go can do Atkins just as easily as if they were doing a different type of eating style that has no restrictions. Atkins allows them to do all of this in one shot.

Whether they need to find food at an airport or stop somewhere on their way from appointment to appointment, they can find Atkins-friendly meals at nearly every restaurant that they visit...and so can you.

It is Fast

Many people who choose to do Atkins do it because of the fast weight loss that they can achieve. Celebrities are put under an immense amount of pressure to lose weight fast. For example, Kim Kardashian needed to lose her baby weight much faster than she put it on. For that reason, she did the Atkins diet. She wanted to be able to lose as much weight possible and that meant that she had to start cutting carbs and fast.

When she was able to cut the carbs out, she started shedding pounds quickly. It is something that celebrities have been doing for ages and something that they will likely continue to do as they work to make sure that they are going to be able to lose weight in the way that they are supposed to. This will be a great way for you to lose weight, too. You just have to make sure that you are going to be able to figure out the right way that weight loss works and the way that you can make sure that you are getting the most out of the experience.

Some celebrities need to lose weight really fast for movie roles. Almost always, they rely on Atkins to be able to lose that weight since it seems to start falling off after they have started the diet. It is a trick that they can use and something that will help them to feel satisfied even when they are losing a huge amount of weight for a role that they are going to be playing.

Chapter 11: Why You Don't Need to Count

The number one benefit of the Atkins diet is that you can lose weight without ever having to count a single calorie or restrict the amount of food that you are eating. This is often one of the biggest reasons that people fail at their diets but it is not something that you will need to deal with if you are doing the Atkins diet. Be sure that you are always trying to make sure that you watch your portions but don't worry about how restricted you are going to be.

Other diets require you to count calories, do complicated math problems to figure out a points system and even eat artificial foods that have had the fat removed from them – Atkins does not. You can eat the Atkins diet in a completely natural way and get your body back to where it was intended to be. This is something that people love about the Atkins diet and something that you will be sure to benefit from when you are working to make sure that your caloric intake is as good as possible. Make sure that you are prepared to eat your favorite foods. The Atkins diet even lets you eat bacon – what other diet can say that?

The only reason you will ever need to check a nutritional fact label is to check and see if a food has any carbs in it. You don't need to worry about the calories in the food or anything else because you will just be watching out for carbs.

Chapter 12: Atkins Recipes

Breakfast

Almond Protein Pancakes

2 oz of whey protein
1/4 ~ cup almond flour
1 ~ tsp baking powder
3 ~ eggs
1/3 cup of cottage cheese

Mix your gelatin and your coconut flour together. Melt your butter and add it into the mixture with the dry ingredients. Stir it up and then add the eggs to it. Make sure that you are mixing it up until there are no clumps in it so that you will not have large pieces or chunks in your pancakes when they are done. Stir in the chives and the bacon gently so that they do not get too mixed up. Pour the mixture into a pan that has butter in it over medium heat. When the pancakes start to bubble, flip them just like you would with real pancakes.

Spicy Omelet

3 ~ links of spicy sausage, chopped into small pieces
2 ~ tbsp. butter that is softened for frying the eggs
3 ~ eggs
1 ~ tsp of water
1 ~ oz of goat cheese
6 ~ leaves of spinach
½ ~ avocado
½ ~ cup of salsa, for the top

Cut your avocado so that it's in pieces. Mix it up with just a little bit of salsa and the spinach. Add the goat cheese. Heat up your pan so that it is on medium heat. Put the butter in and allow it to start to melt. Put the eggs into the pan. Put your avocado mixture in with the eggs and then put the chorizo on top of all of it. This will allow you to make sure that you are going to be able to make the ingredients. Once the egg starts to set up, fold it over and continue to cook it until it is fully cooked.

Lunch

Chicken Caesar Wrap

4 ~ leaves of lettuce
½ ~ of an avocado
½ ~ of a cup of parmesan
1 ~ cooked chicken cubed up
3 ~ tbsp. Caesar dressing, carb free

Lay your lettuce leaves out so that they are in a line and they are like tortillas that you would normally put into a wrap. Place the dressing on top of the lettuce. Add the parmesan cheese on top of that. Put the cubed chicken on top of all of that. Top with the avocado. Wrap the lettuce up like a tortilla and secure with a toothpick so that they do not come unwrapped.

Tuna Salad

1 ~ cup mayonnaise
1 ~ tin of tuna that is packed in oil
1 ~ tsp of mustard
1 ~ tsp of salt
1 ~ tsp of pepper
½ ~ tsp of paprika

Mix all of your ingredients up and stir well to make sure that you are breaking up all of the pieces of tuna. Be sure that you stir it and there are no small pieces of the spices that have become clumped together. After you have completely stirred it, you can put it aside and put it in the fridge as a snack on its own or as a lunch wrapped up in a piece of lettuce. You can also add some chopped boiled eggs to the salad to add some extra texture to it.

Barbecue Salad

2 ~ cups of lettuce chopped up
1 ~ cup of cooked chicken in cubes
½ ~ tbsp. of barbecue sauce
½ ~ tbsp. of ranch sauce
½ ~ cup of tomato that is chopped up
2 ~ boiled eggs that are cut into cubes
4 ~ slices of bacon that are crumbled into pieces or,

alternatively, bacon crumbles (be sure to get real and not imitation as those contain carbs)

Mix the ingredients all together except for the ranch dressing and shake to make sure that they are well combined. You can then top with the ranch dressing and eat or simply toss again to help it mix up with the other ingredients. If you are past the first stage of Atkins, you can also add black beans to the salad to give it some extra substance and to make it taste better but do not add too many of the beans or do it before you're past phase 1 because they have (healthy) carbs that are in them.

Dinner

Cheeseburger Casserole

1 ~ lb of ground beef that is cooked completely
2 ~ cups of cheddar cheese
1 ~ tbsp. of tomato paste
6 ~ eggs that are mixed up completely
½ ~ cup of pickles that are chopped up into small pieces

Put ground beef in casserole dish. Stir in the cheddar cheese. Mix the tomato paste with it. You can also put a small amount of cream in the tomato paste to make it easier to mix up. Blend in the pickles with this part of the mixture. When this is blended up, mix up the eggs with it and then grease a large pan with butter or coconut oil. Pour the mixture into the pan and bake in your oven at 400 degrees for anywhere between 25 and 40 minutes. When it is done, it will not be liquid but it will still be somewhat jiggly so that you can continue to make sure that it is fully cooked. You can add any of your favorite burger toppings to the casserole and then top with some extra cheddar cheese on the top. Switch for pepper jack for a spicy flavor.

Cordon Bleu Casserole

1 ~ lb of chicken breast that is fully cooked and cut into small pieces
½ ~ lb of ham that is chopped up into small pieces
½ ~ lb of swiss cheese
1 ~ box of cream cheese that is softened
1 ~ tbsp. of Dijon mustard

1 ~ tsp of white wine
1 ~ tsp salt
1 ~ tsp pepper

Create the sauce for the recipe with the last five ingredients that are listed in this recipe. Mix up the chicken with the ham and then stir them up so that they are mixed in with the rest of the ingredients and are coated in the sauce that you are going to be able to use. Top it off with the swiss cheese. Heat your oven up to 350 degrees and cook the casserole for 20-30 minutes or until the cheese is bubbly on top. Once it has melted, turn your broiler on for a minute or two and then allow it to get browned on the top. Serve with green beans or any other type of vegetable that is Atkins friendly and does not have any carbs in it.

Steak Bites

1 ~ large sirloin steak that is cut into cube sized pieces
½ ~ c soy sauce
½ ~ tbsp. of minced garlic
1 ~ tsp onion powder
1 ~ tsp of sweetener
1 ~ tsp of salt
1 ~ tsp of pepper
½ ~ c of Worcestershire sauce
1 ~ tsp parsley
1 ~ tsp of basil

Soak your steak cubes in the sauce that you have just created with the rest of the ingredients. Allow it to soak for a few hours or overnight for the best flavor possible. After the steak is completely marinated, put 1 tbsp of butter in a pan and heat it up over high heat. Do not allow it to burn. Reduce it to a low heat and then simmer the steak bites to cook for about 15 minutes or until they are completely cooked through to your desired doneness. When they are done, serve them with fried peppers and onions or with any of your favorite vegetables.

Snacks

Caribbean Meatballs

1 ~ package of meatballs with no carbs (or, if you can't find any, make your own)
1 ~ tbsp. jerk seasoning
1 ~ tsp of pepper
1 ~ tsp of salt

Mix all of the ingredients together and place them into a slow cooker. Allow them to cook for 4 hours on high or until the meatballs are tender and completely cooked. You can put the meatballs out on a plate to eat them right away or you can put them in the refrigerator to save for later on. Serve them with soy sauce or teriyaki sauce for an extra kick to the flavor of them.

Cocktail Wieners

1 ~ jar of chili sauce
1 ~ jar of sugar-free grape jelly
2 ~ packages of Lil' smokies

Mix all of the ingredients up together and put them in a small crockpot. Heat them up on low for 4 hours or simply put them on the warm function of your slow cooker. Be sure that you are stirring them every once in a while so that they do not become clumped together.

Stuffed Mushrooms

1 ~ pint of mushrooms that are cremini
1 ~ box of cream cheese
½ ~ c of real bacon bits
1 ~ tbsp. of chives or chopped green onions

Take the caps off of the mushrooms and clean them. Allow the cream cheese to soften up so that you can mix it up. Mix the bacon bits, the green onions, and the cream cheese together so that they are all well blended up. Lay the mushrooms out with the wells facing up where the stems were at. Stuff the mushrooms with the cream cheese mixture that you just created and then put them in the oven at 350 degrees for 15-25 minutes or until they start to get soft.

Crab Cakes

1 lb of crab meat
1 scallion finely chopped
1 cup of mayonnaise
3tbsp of finely chopped parsley
½ a tsp of any seasoning of your choice
1 cup of low carb bread crumbs mix
3 tbsp of oil

Heat up your oil on medium high temperature. Add in scallions and bell pepper and sauté until softened. Now transfer the sauté mixture into a large bowl. Add the crab meat, mayo, parsley and seasoning into the bowl. Mix with a fork, but be sure not to over mix. Get a 1/3 cup measuring cup and place breadcrumbs into it. Fill the measuring cup with crab mixture and sprinkle more bread crumbs. Invert crab mixture onto a baking sheet and cover with plastic wrap and refrigerate for at least an hour. Then heat oil in skillet and cook crab cakes for 3 to 4minutes or until golden brown.

Conclusion

Thanks for making it through to the end of *Atkins Diet*. Let's hope it was informative and able to provide you with all of the tools you need to achieve your goals of losing weight and getting that body you've always wanted.

The next step is to stop eating carbs – it's as simple as that.

Finally, if you found this book useful in any way, a review on Amazon is always appreciated!

DISCLAIMER: Please don't panic if you don't see results immediately. It takes a bit of time for your body to enter ketosis and reprogram itself to use stored fat for fuel instead of carbohydrates. Every individual's body is different.